Health Mentor in a Book

9-day protocol reset

How one can Apply these daily tips to change health statuses.

Some read and get the information and say, "Yes, I have good knowledge of health information and execute in pain.

And

Those who can say "Yes I have firsthand application and experience of this knowledge."

"Change my expectations and I will change my conditions."

-Tony Robins

Author: *Suzette Persaud*

My wellness

Table of Contents

Send your Questions to infinitsuccess911@gmail.com --------------

PREFACE

<u>**"Mentor in a book"**</u>, true assistance at your fingertips.

Thomas Edison "No one can overcome a health problem using the same mindset that created the problem."

DISCLAIMER

The information in this book is not intended to diagnose, treat, cure, or prevent any conditions or diseases. The reader understands Mentor in a book and the information within is not a substitute for consultation with a licensed practitioner. The use of this book implies your acceptance of the disclaimer.

<u>level 1 detox</u>

Morning

- smoothie or smoothie bowl
- fruits or fruit-only salad
- Fresh Coconut water
- apples, mangoes, pears
- bananas etc
- berries- any kind
- MELONS-water melon (seeded)
- cantaloupe, honey dew, papaya, casaba, canary
- herbal teas Dandelion root
- Moringa

LUNCH

- green salads, cucumbers, alfalfa sprouts, tomatoes, avocados

- fruit salad, fruit smoothie.

- Moringa

Dinner

- small portion of steamed veggies

- veggie soup, steamed squash, pumpkin, zucchini.

- Avocado

- Dandelion root herbal tea

<u>Snack</u>

Raw fruit or raw fruit juice

level 2 detox

— 8 —

morning

- raw fruit juice (Berries only any kind)

- fruits citrus any kind

- herbal teas (see list below)

- apples, mangoes, pears bananas etc.

- melons any kind (cantaloupe, honey dew, papaya, casaba, canary etc)

- coconut water etc.

Lunch

- veggie soup broth (no solids)

- herbs (thyme, oregano, parsley, Moringa) etc.

Dinner

- raw fruits, berries or melons any kind

- raw fruit juice only no smoothie, no greens

EXITING A FAST

Extreme caution is to be taken when exiting a fast.

<u>Level 1 Detox Exit.</u>

<u>**Do Not**</u>   carbs, NO meat, NO eggs, NO dairy, NO

Cheese NO

Greens or green salad.

<u>DO'S</u>   smoothies, vegetable soups, and broth,

and eat

raw fruits, and ground fruits,

DO NOT

1. don't drink just any liquid.
2. don't eat any solids
3. don't eat any salads
4. NO SOLID FOODS TO BE INGESTED

<u>DO'S</u>

1. drink pure coconut water drink slowly no gulping and only ¼ cup at a time
2. drink watermelon juice, not the fibers just pure juice ¼ cup at a time.
3. Drink pure cucumber juice with no fibers
4. Drink melon juice only with no fibers
5. Drink pure grape juice with no fibers

Of all the above dos, choose only one type of juice for the day and drink as needed, starting with ¼ cups the first hour, then ½ cups, and 3 hours later ¾ cups. Then, work yourself to 1 full cup for the day.

- Day **2** follows the same steps as day one (no solids.)
- Do drink any of the above fruit juice in any order
- Day **3**: Continue with a smoothie, fruit, or fruit salad.

I recommend leafy green salads on day 4 level 1 detox post protocol with all other regular salads except <u>No meat, fish, or eggs absolutely NO FLESH.</u>

After your long days of abstinence, you are now here in the center of "SELF" where there are 3 paths to choose from this outcome of your short journey.

1. Frugivore lifestyle 90/10
2. Vegetarian conscientious lifestyle 50/50 vegetables and fruits some eggs or cooked fish (no sushi)
3. S.A.D lifestyle 50/50 grains, vegetables, meat flesh, manmade meat, juice, wine, liquor, etc.

Without mentioning the new age "vegan" this lifestyle is restrictive to imitating foods without thought of the soul, being the physical state of health.

I.   If the choice is 2 vegetarian 50/50 then detox level one is recommended once every month for 6-9 days protocol

II.   Choice number 3. S.A.D here is level 4 detox and, in most cases, depending on where you are in your circumstances health-wise

III.

Level 4 once every month or level 4 with consultation from a professional or recommended follow-up with a doctor along with level 4 detox combination.

<u>overview</u>

Getting started on a wellness protocol for 6 days takes some preparation of the mind.

The 6-day protocol is truly **9 days** considering that magical moment of exiting a restricted diet that needs **3 days** before integrating into your choice of a "normal" daily dietary routine.

Let's get started on a sample protocol for 6 days which most individuals can use with or without any restrictions. However, it is advisable to check in with your health care provider to get your blood levels checked and ask for a bit of guidance. This protocol will improve gut health and improve heart wellness and brain due to their deep connection.

As long as your healthcare provider approves, they may or may not work with you all depending on your health status so please seek healthcare professionals' help in this regard.

6-day protocol with 3-day exit plan

Eat nothing for the full 6 days of your normal diet, except for what is specified in this protocol.

This protocol consists of fruits, vegetables, herbs, and vitamins. You can use this as a guide in your own journey.

Many of the concerns will be "Fruits', oh the "SUGAR IN FRUITS".

Remember simple sugars are the MONOSACCHARIDES:

- Glucose from vegetables which contains 6 carbon bonds known as hexoses.
- Fructose from fruits which contains 6 carbon bonds known as hexoses.
- Galactose-from milk(this is for infants only)with 6 carbon bonds known as hexoses

- (RNA)Ribose -from fruits & vegetables this contains 5 carbon bonds known as pentoses.
- (DNA)Deoxyribose-also from fruits and vegetables with 5 carbons known as pentoses

These are simple sugars with no fermentation needed, fruits have high astringent and antioxidant properties, help blood sugar conditions, the pancreas, and other gastric, gut health issues.

Fruits are highly electrical and is superior for our wellness

Vegetables are much lower electrically in detoxification and bring the body to wellness.

Now let's dive right into this 6-day protocol guide.

Protocol guide

eat nothing for the full 6 days other than as specified during this protocol if you are experiencing extreme hunger you may sip on specified herbal teas or broth or specified fruit juice plenty of liquid is required for this specific protocol.

Mentor protocol

Level 1 detox

Day 1:

dandelion root tea no milk no sweeteners

The fruit smoothie should be papaya with seeds at least one glass every day For six days blend and drink.

Or

Fruit smoothie with fruits of your choice added One tablespoon of moringa powder. For sweetener add 1 to 2 tablespoons of xylitol sugar.

3 magnesium L-threonate three times daily for 6 days.

Pau D' arco 2 capsules daily

black walnut and Wormwood 2 capsules daily

green walnut and Wormwood 2 capsules daily

oregano with black seed oil 2 capsules daily

1 adrenal glandular

3 bone n' marrow glandular (freeze-dried) twice daily

1 capsule of cayenne pepper with one full glass of fresh Fruit juice

Drink as much fruit juice as needed fresh fruit juice throughout the day nothing solid to be ingested.

Mentor protocol

<u>Day 2</u>

fruit smoothie with fruits of your choice add 1 tablespoon of moringa powder and for sweetener add 1 to 2 tablespoon xylitol sugar.

Or

fruit smoothies should be papaya with seeds at least one glass every day for six days blend and drink (distilled water preferably)

3 magnesium L-threonate three times daily for 6 days.

Pau D' arco 2 capsules daily

black walnuts & Wormwood 2 capsules daily

green walnut & Wormwood 2 capsules daily

oregano with black seed oil 2 capsules daily

1 adrenal glandular (freeze-dried)

3 bone and marrow glandular twice daily

1 capsule of cayenne pepper with one full glass of fresh fruit juice.

Drink as much fruit juice as needed.

fresh fruit juice throughout the day nothing solid to be ingested.

Dandelion root tea or any other herbal tea of choice (no sweetener added).

mentor protocol

Day 3

dandelion root tea or any herbal tea of choice, no milk no sweetener

fruit smoothie of choice, one tablespoon of moringa added, for sweetener use 2 tablespoons of xylitol sugar.

3 magnesium L -threonate three times daily for six days

Pau D' arco 2 capsules daily

black walnut and Wormwood 2 capsules daily

green walnut and Wormwood 2 capsules daily

Oregano with black seed oil 2 capsule capsules daily

1 adrenal glandular

3 bone & marrow glandular twice daily

one capsule of cayenne pepper with one full glass of fresh fruit juice

drink as much fruit juice as needed fresh fruit juice throughout the day nothing solid to be ingested.

Mentor protocol

Day 4

Dandelion tea or any herbal tea of choice

Fruit smoothie of choice add one tablespoon of moringa powder for sweetener add 1 to 2 tablespoons of xylitol sugar.

3 magnesium L -threonate three times daily for 6 days

Paul D' arco 2 capsules daily

black walnut & Wormwood 2 capsules daily

green walnut & Wormwood 2 capsules daily

oregano and black seed oil 2 capsules daily

1 adrenal glandular

1 capsule of cayenne pepper with one full glass of fresh fruit juice

drink as much fruit juice as needed fresh fruit juice throughout the day nothing solid to be ingested

Mentor protocol

<u>Day 5</u>

herbal tea of choice (distilled water preferably)

fruit smoothie with fruits of your choice add 1 tablespoon of moringa powder, for sweetener add 1 to 2 tablespoon of xylitol sugar.

3 magnesium L-threonate three times daily for 6 days

Paul D' arco 2 capsules daily

black walnut and Wormwood 2 capsules daily

green walnut and Wormwood 2 capsules daily

oregano with black seed oil 2 capsules daily

one adrenal glandular

3 bone n' marrow glandular twice daily

1 capsule of cayenne pepper with one full glass of fresh fruit juice

drink as much fruit juice as needed, fresh fruit juice throughout the day nothing solid to be ingested.

My wellness

Mentor protocol

<u>Day 6</u>

Dandelion root tea or any herbal tea of your choice (distill preferably)

Fruit smoothie with fruits of your choice add 1 tablespoon of moringa powder,

1 for sweetener add 1 to **2** tablespoons of xylitol sugar.

3 magnesium L -threonate three times daily for **6** days

Paul D' arco capsules **2** daily

black walnut n' Wormwood **2** capsules daily

green walnuts n' Wormwood **2** capsules daily

oregano with black seed oil **2** capsules daily

1 adrenal glandular

three bone n' marrow glandular twice daily

1 capsule of cayenne pepper with 1 full glass of fresh fruit juice

drink as much fruit juice as needed fresh fruit juice throughout the day nothing solid to be ingested.

Break or Exit fast

WOW! If you followed along and made it to the end of this **6**-day fruit juice Protocol

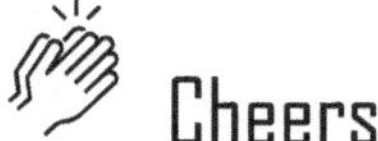 Cheers!

Preparing the mind for this **6**-day journey and sticking to the protocol is a huge accomplishment. Now, breaking a fast is even more important, and here is a rule to follow for a **6**-day juice fast **2** full days of continued fresh fruit juice and eating only fresh fruits (fresh and raw: all melons and berries no exceptions).

Day **3** fruit smoothies, fresh fruit juice, eating more fruits and fruits of choice.

Recap: post 6day fruit juice fasting

3 days of fresh fruit juice, fresh raw fruits, fruit salad, melons all types of melon, and berries.

Post fruit fast add vegetable broth, and cucumber zucchini lightly sauté salad. At this point after your journey, you now get to decide what is next.

My wellness

It's very important to keep the bowels moving during any juice fast. Keeping bowels moving during these times is not always possible.

Self-observation

Day1	**Day2**

<table>
<tr><td>Day3</td><td>Day4</td></tr>
<tr><td>

</td><td></td></tr>
</table>

Self-check to follow up each day.

My observation 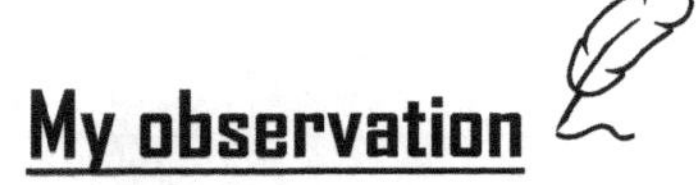

Day5	Day6

self-check to follow up each day

My wellness

Notes:

Starch is very hard to digest and its mucus-forming

limit your: bread, cereal corn potato intake.

Notes:

Vegetables are the muscular-skeletal foods

Notes:

Fruits are our energy, antioxidant, and astringent nourishment.

One day at a time for 6 days while observing the body, the inner self, and the mind.

If you make it to the full 6-9 day the door to self is open and ready to continue further down the path to wellness.

Allow our food to be our medicine, as the great father Hippocrates of medicine once said.

To go deeper into detoxification and protocol please consult a trained professional to help guide you, especially if your body is in a much deeper state and needs much closer care and guidance to wellness.

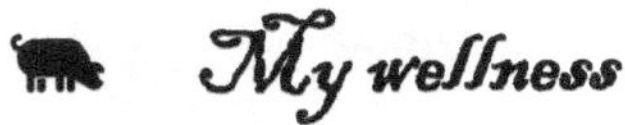

Bonus:

Herbal teas for quick remedies:

Anemia – Dandelion Root tea, <u>use</u> (distilled water for brewing)

Asthma - Mullein, Eucalyptus, and mugwort leaves use Distilled water.

Headache -Valerian and chamomile (do not use while operating any machinery or driving drink only when ready to lay down and rest**)**

Glandular

Adrenal glandular plays a vital role in strengthening the adrenal glands which has an important role with every cell in our body.

Bone marrow glandular is like the stem cell in our system. Contains essential nourishments, collagen, the substance needed to build and repair and maintain our bones and connective tissues.

The glandular is there to help empower the cells in the body from its weak state. Glandular were designed and have been used for temporary short-term restoration of weakened states in the body.

My Wellness

Bonus:

Diabetic 14-day tips

Exercise, to begin, needs an intensity of 10,15, 25 to 30 minutes of workout first thing in the morning following a glass of pure coconut water for hydration of cells.

If no coconut water is available drink melon drink fresh melon blended in distilled water or juice of pure melon of any type.

Stay away from wheat dairy-bleached flour no refined sugar, no honey no agave, no maple, no caffeine.

Use xylitol sugar only,

need real cow butter ghee /Tallow glandular

avocado oil, lots of avocado fruit, olive oil sesame oil

lots of nuts and seeds (easy with the cashew seed) stay away from **peanut**

Lunch should be at noon when the sun is high; Eat a large portion.

quinoa, Kamut green salads/vegetables

no meat, chicken, duck, goat, lamb, pork, beef, or shellfish.

Bonus insight from https://pubmed.ncbi.nlm.nih.gov/

Does high-dose vitamin D supplementation impact insulin resistance and risk of development of diabetes in patients with pre-diabetes? A double-blind randomized clinical trial

Mahtab Niroomand [1], Akbar Fotouhi [2], Navid Irannejad [3], Farhad Hosseinpanah [4]
Affiliations Expand

- PMID: 30583032

- DOI: 10.1016/j.diabres.2018.12.008

Abstract

Aims: The aim of this study is to evaluate the effect of high-dose vitamin D on insulin sensitivity and the risk of progression to diabetes.

Methods: In this double-blind, placebo-controlled randomized clinical trial adults with pre-diabetes and vitamin D deficiency were randomly assigned to either vitamin D$_3$ or placebo. Fasting plasma glucose (FPG), 2-h oral glucose tolerance test plasma glucose (OGTT PG), Homeostatic Model Assessment of Insulin Resistance (HOMA-IR), and the rate of progression of glucose tolerance was compared.

Results: A total of 162 patients were randomized, from which 83 finished the 6-month follow-up (44 in intervention group and 39 in control group). In 6 months, serum 25-hydroxyvitamin D levels were significantly higher in the intervention group (36 ng/ml vs 16 ng/ml, P value < 0.001). There was no significant difference between FPG or 2H-OGTT PG in two groups. HOMA-IR score was significantly lower in the vitamin D group (2.6 vs. 3.1; P value = 0.04). The rate of progression toward diabetes was significantly lower in the intervention group (28% vs. 3%; P value = 0.002).

Conclusions: In patients with pre-diabetes and hypovitaminosis D, high dose vitamin D improves insulin sensitivity and decreases risk of progression toward diabetes.

Keywords: Diabetes; Insulin resistance; Prevention; Vitamin D.

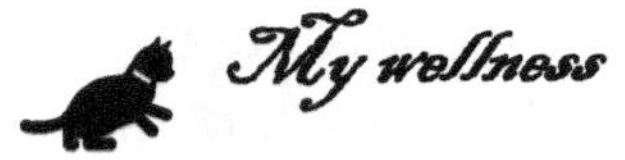

Questions and Answers

Q: Can I add ginger to my juices?

A: freshly squeezed is ideal

Q: Is this safe while on medication?

A: first follow your medication instruction and talk to your doctor begin.

Q: What if I become malnourished?

A: Great question always consults with your doctor if suffering medical issues   before proceeding.

level 1 protocol for six days done right will nourish your cells and rejuvenate your mind, body, emotion and soul.

Q: I am anemic, can I go on this detox protocol?

A: Yes, being anemic is due to weak adrenal, start with the level 1 detox protocol take follow the protocol as directed also great way to add some burdock, Irish sea moss, Yellow dock and use the adrenal glandular.

Q: What about veggies why is it off the protocol

A: vegetables are not astringent and therefore not great detoxifier; Veggies are muscle builder

My wellness protocol

Resources for glandular

Adrenal glandular

Bone marrow glandular

https://liveancestral.com/ancestral-supplements-adrenal/

— 33 —

My wellness thoughts

— 34 —

My wellness thoughts

My wellness

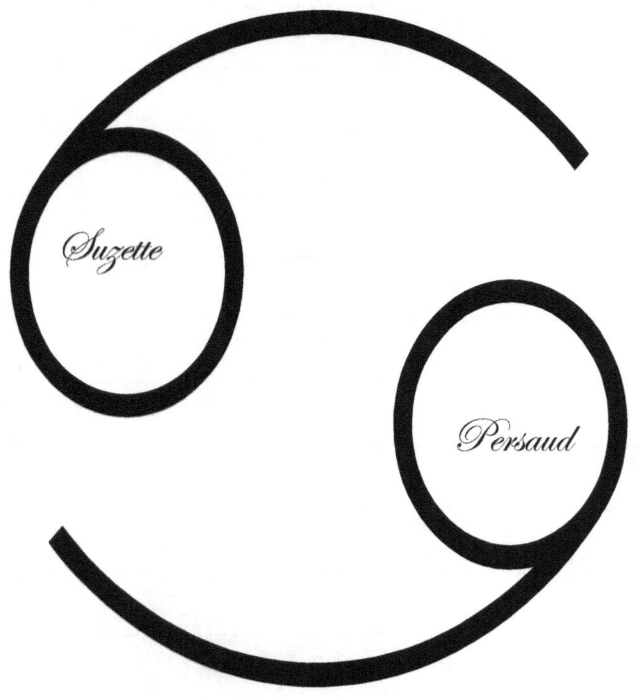

Suzette
Persaud

Self-observation

It does not matter what condition of health you are in.

your journey to wellness ✓

What an incredible joy in your life.

Thank You

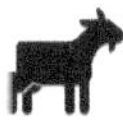